Mediterranean Diet

The Alternative bound to be Life-changing

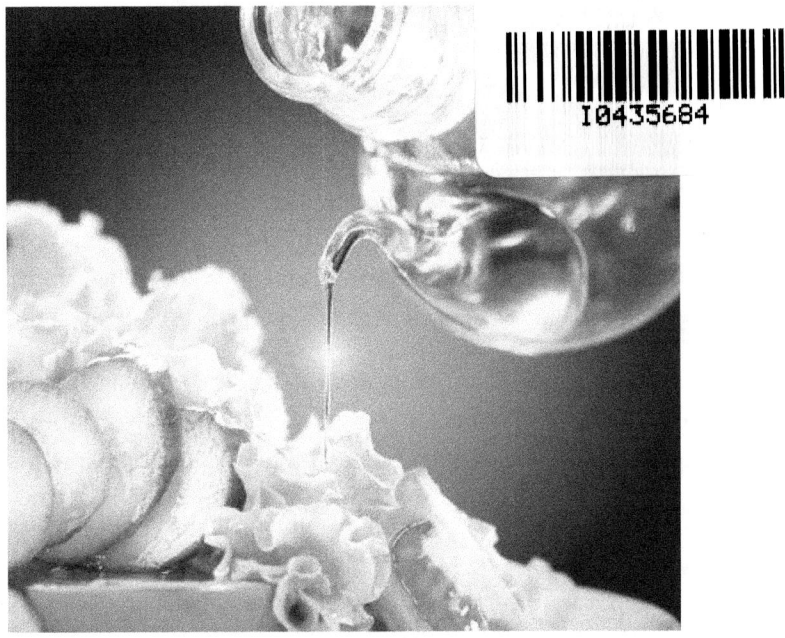

Health Learning Series

M. Usman
Mendon Cottage Books

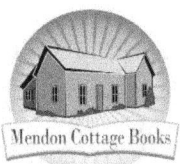

JD-Biz Publishing

Disclaimer

The information is this book is provided for informational purposes only. It is not intended to be used and medical advice or a substitute for proper medical treatment by a qualified health care provider. The information is believed to be accurate as presented based on research by the author.

The contents have not been evaluated by the U.S. Food and Drug Administration or any other Government or Health Organization and the contents in this book are not to be used to treat cure or prevent disease.

The author or publisher is not responsible for the use or safety of any diet, procedure or treatment mentioned in this book. The author or publisher is not responsible for errors or omissions that may exist.

Warning

The Book is for informational purposes only and before taking on any diet, treatment or medical procedure, it is recommended to consult with your primary health care provider.

Our books are available at

1. Amazon.com
2. Barnes and Noble
3. Itunes
4. Kobo
5. Smashwords
6. Google Play Books

Table of Contents

Prelude

The Mediterranean diet is a way of eating that is followed by people living in countries surrounding the Mediterranean region. The diet is just like any other personalized diet in the world and has nothing fancy in it. The population of these regions consume it like Americans consume pizzas, Indians consume vegetables, or Chinese consume rice. But, the diet has gained wide spread attention due to the great number of health benefits it brings for a person. The diet is not something to follow forcefully but something that you will adjust to as time passes. Imagine replacing your current diet regimen, with a healthier one and the transition will become much easier. The diet comes with a multitude of benefits which can be evidently seen in the people of the Mediterranean region. The benefits include reduction of heart disease risk, protection against Parkinson's, Alzheimer's, and improvement of the immunity system as well as the gastrointestinal one.

More is explained in the following chapter so read on and get ready to change your life for the better.

Mediterranean Diet Starters

Chapter 1: Overview

The word Mediterranean isn't an unheard one. We encounter it all the time in newspapers, films and TV shows, but we seldom hear it in combination with the word diet or nutrition. Some of you might have, but the majority of the population knows this region only for its great tourist resorts. This mindset is about to change.

The world of diets is a just like space; it keeps on expanding. Recently the popularity of natural diets has skyrocketed and dwarfed the artificial ones due to the lackluster and sometimes harmful performance by the latter. A little journey into this world shows that the number of diets existing in the world is increasing at an exponential rate, each one marketed in a manner to work out your weaknesses. Many people have actually fallen into this trap and have lost more than they could gain. Thus, the world is now shifting towards the better side of the bargain which includes efficient, natural, and most importantly, health promoting natural diets, just like the Mediterranean one.

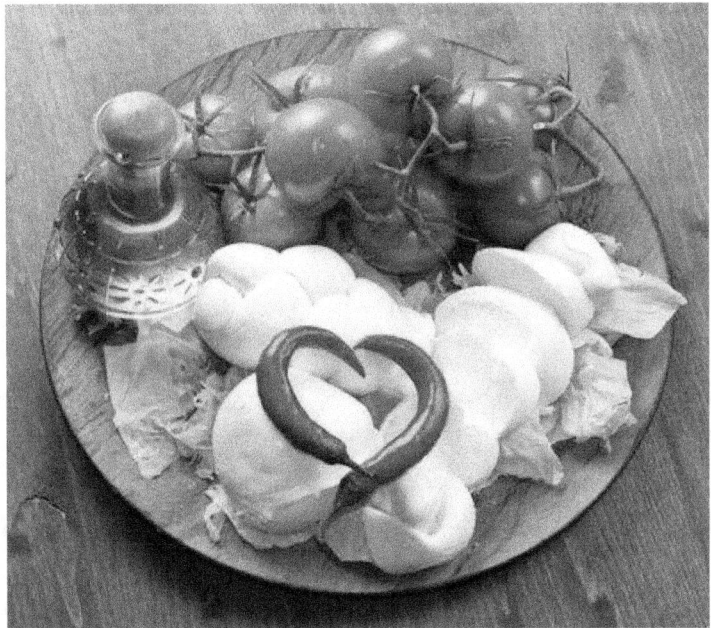

Shortly after the Second World War, Ancel Keys, along with his colleagues, developed interest into the intriguing Mediterranean diet. They organized a study that aimed to find out the impacts of the diet on humans. The study was known as the Seven Countries Study and went on for a long time, targeting a great number of individuals from many countries. 13,000 middle aged men were chosen for the study from US, Italy, Greece, Japan, Finland, Netherlands and Yugoslavia. An examination of the individuals revealed that Cretan men had the lowest death rates from heart disease even though they consumed significant amounts of fat. Furthermore, it was found that inclusion of the Mediterranean diet in one's food significantly lowered the risk of cardiovascular disease. In the years following this study, the diet gained widespread attention from both the public, as well as, medical experts, but it wasn't until the 90s that the diet became truly popular. Since then, the diet has become a part of the mainstream and many people today have totally shifted their eating patterns to get the best of the diet.

Chapter 2: What to Eat?

The Mediterranean diet is a UNESCO recognized diet pattern which focuses primarily on high consumption of foods like legumes, brown cereals, vegetables, fruits and olive oil. Moreover, a significant portion of the diet consists of fish and other sea food along with probiotic dairy products like yogurt and cheese. That's not all; the Mediterranean diet is not an expensive one and can easily merge into your kitchen budget without raising a lot of eyebrows! A very general overview of the diet's main components is as follows:

1.   **Vegetables**:

Vegetables are an integral part of the Mediterranean cuisine primarily due to the freshness and abundant resource of nutrients they add to a meal. From a plate of sliced tomatoes seasoned with olive oil and cheese to complex salad combinations, stews pizzas, and roasted products, vegetables are a prime ingredient in any Mediterranean food plan.

2.   **Meat:**

Some of you might have been astonished after reading this word in a healthy diet. It must be known that meat is not the root cause of every disease developed in a person. It's time to change the way you perceive meat and its effects. If small strips of beef, chicken or lamb are consumed along with fresh vegetables and yogurt, many harmful effects of meat can be eliminated.

3.   **Dairy products:**

Greek cheese and yogurt are two dairy products not unheard of. They are loaded with several benefits primarily for the gastrointestinal tract. These products contain probiotics that relieve the body of many of the after effects of anti-biotics or bad bacteria, primarily in the digestive tract.

4.   **Seafood:**

Fish are a host to several minerals, nutrients and compounds, the most vital of which is the omega-3 fatty acid. Fish like herring, salmon, tuna and sardines are rich in this particular fatty acid which has benefits for the heart as well as the brain.

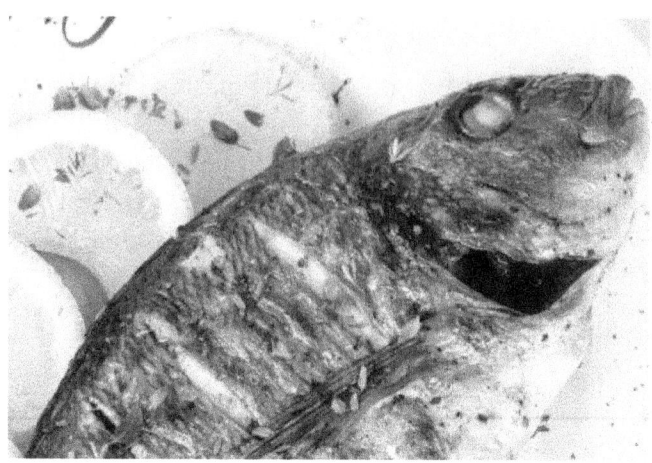

5. Good fats:

The Mediterranean diet is rich in fats as well. These fats are not harmful to the body, but actually help the body regain its proper form. Fats obtained from nuts, seeds, olives, peanuts and avocados are essential for proper skin, vascular and immunity-boosting functions.

6. Whole Grains:

Whole grains are a class of foods that are respected around the whole world, irrespective of the region. Whole grains are rich in nutrients that are lost otherwise when the grains are processed; this gives them a fuller taste along with an additional serving of fiber which keeps you satiated for hours. Traditional Mediterranean grains include brown, black and red rice, barley, bulgur, faro and products made out of whole grains.

7. Fruit:

It's best if you choose fresh fruits for dessert! The Mediterranean cuisine allows you to choose from a variety of fruits including figs, oranges, grapes, apples, pomegranates, etc. You can also use Mediterranean ingredients to prepare a sweet dish if you like.

When all of these foods are eaten in combination and become a part of a person's diet, they bring great improvement in the person's overall health profile. A number of studies have showed that the diet actually proves beneficial for the body and a person following the specific pattern can be protected against damage done to the heart, brain, intestines and immunity system.

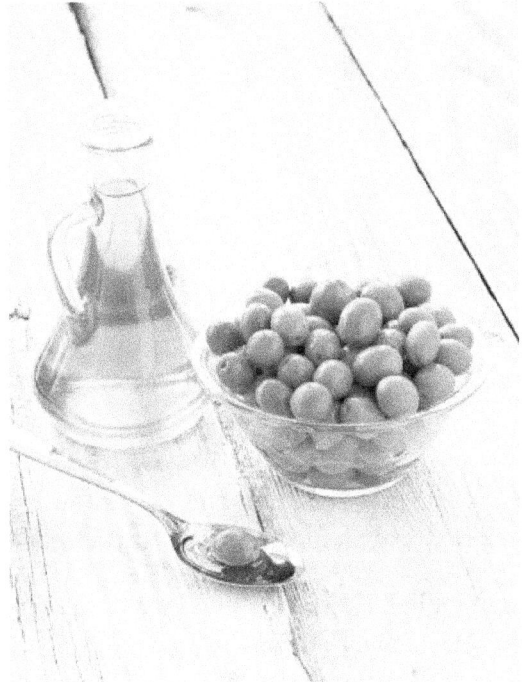

Chapter 3: Mediterranean Diet Pyramid

As interest in the diet reached its peak, a group of researchers at the Harvard School of Public Health and the European Office of WHO presented the Diet along with a clever way to understand it, visually. The graphic approach was known as the Mediterranean Diet Pyramid which to this day, has become a universally accepted way for developing eating patterns comprising of Mediterranean cuisine. It is widely used by educators, consumers and medical experts to implement better eating habits.

The pyramid was developed using the latest medical findings with respect to the diet using studies, researches and work of various medical professionals. It was found that the Mediterranean people followed a diet pattern that more or less remained unchanged throughout history. The main constituents of the diet have already been given in the previous chapter but the amount of each food item is also a matter of importance.

i.   Food obtained from plants, to be eaten in abundance. These foods included vegetables, fruits, breads, beans, nuts and seeds.

ii.   Little reliance on processed foods no matter how little they are; fresh and locally grown foods must be maximized in one's diet.

iii.   Inclusion of fat in the diet, but only from olive oil, butter and margarine. The amount of fat consumed must be ranging from 25 to 35 percent of energy; saturated fat up to 8 percent of energy.

iv.   Low to moderate consumption of dairy products like cheese, yogurt and milk.

v.   Consumption of moderate amounts of fish as well as poultry, twice a week; studies have showed that consumption of 7 eggs per week can prove beneficial for the body.

vi.   For dessert, consumption of fresh fruit, a few times a week; the fruit may be served either with sugar or honey.

vii.   Red meat, only a few times a month; its consumption should be limited to 340 to 450 grams a month. The lean versions of the meat are more preferred over the simple ones.

viii.   Moderate consumption of wine, usually with meals; this accounts for 1-2 glasses a day for men whereas women should consume only 1 glass.

ix.   All of the above, along with physical activity. The physical activity must not always include running, swimming or weight-lifting, but simply any kind of activity will improve the body's metabolism.

It should be known that the pyramid was not set in stone, but the Advisory board of the pyramid makes occasional changes to its contents. The latest feature of the pyramid includes herbs and spices in its list of allowed foods. The decision was made by the board based on both the health and culinary benefits the spices added to the meal.

Health Benefits

Chapter # 1: Cardiovascular Benefits

Heart disease, be it of any type is, becoming a great source of worry for people of all ages. The risk of being vulnerable to any cardiovascular ailment is increasing day by day and is greatly influenced by what a person consumes throughout the day. In a nutshell, heart disease is a general term used for any type of disease, ailment or condition that affects the heart. Cardiovascular is a term that is used when the blood vessels are also affected in addition to the heart. The WHO states that heart disease is the leading striker of death in many countries.

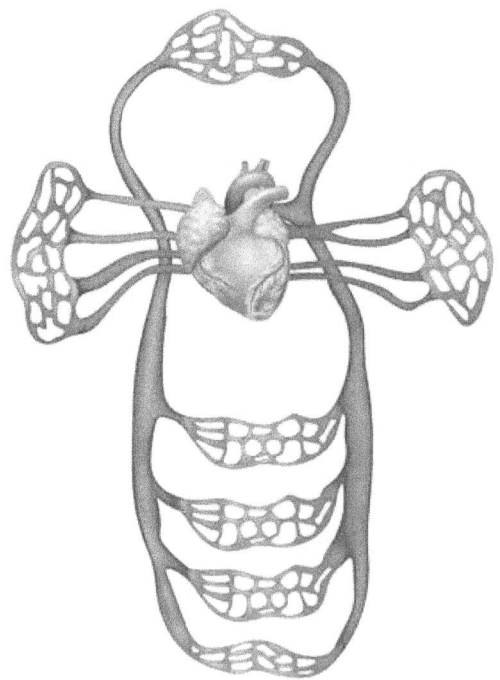

Now researchers have found that the Mediterranean Diet has positive implications on a person's anatomy and especially helps deal with the risk of coronary heart disease. Researchers at the McMaster University evaluated over 200 studies related to dietary patterns and coronary heart disease; the studies were conducted between 1950 and 2007 in the US, Europe and Asia.

The final paper was published in the April 13th issue of Archives of Internal Medicine.

The study was able to show that when certain food groups and/or dietary patterns were followed by an individual, he/she was less exposed to the risk of cardiovascular diseases. These dietary patterns are usually incorporated the nutritional goodness of fruits, vegetables, olive oil, nuts, a little red meat, fish and some wine. Almost all of the patterns were similar to the Mediterranean diet. To further highlight the icing on the cake, it was found that Transfats and foods with a high glycemic index were harmful for the heart.

The researchers stressed the fact that heart diseases were being caused due to lack of attention being paid towards one's diet. Most people are so busy in their life that they actually forget about their health and the significance of an overall diet. The word "overall" needs to be emphasized upon as people must know the advantage of a complete diet like the Mediterranean diet. The researchers stated that whenever they encountered individuals who feasted upon the diet, they noticed a lighter cardiovascular-disease footprint.

Chapter 2: Diabetes

Diabetes is a term to that is familiar to everyone. It is known to doctors by the name of diabetes mellitus and is a group of metabolic imbalances that are characterized by, high blood sugar, inadequate insulin production or irresponsive body cells. The most common symptoms of diabetes include intermittent urination and increasing thirst and hunger. In 2013 it was estimated that over 382 million people throughout the world, were plagued by the disease.

There are two type of diabetes, type 1 and type 2. Type 1 diabetes occurs when the body ceases to produce insulin. Almost 10% cases of diabetes are type 1. A type 1 patient can overcome his/her problem by incorporating a healthy diet, ample exercise and dropping practices like drug abuse, smoking, etc. A type 2 patient however suffers from improper insulin production. Type 2 diabetes can be controlled but can never be eliminated; still the symptoms can be checked to such a level that the person can lead an almost normal life.

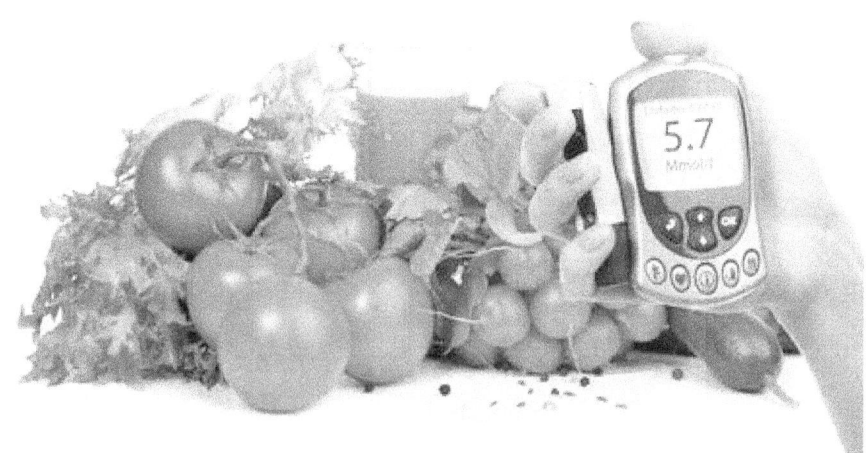

A study published in the 2008 edition of BMJ reported that the Mediterranean diet, rich in fruits, nuts, vegetables, olive oil, etc. can effectively deal with the onset of type-2 diabetes. Previous researches had shown that the original Mediterranean diet could provide protection against cardiovascular conditions, but the protective effect against diabetes was still unknown. To investigate the link between the diet and diabetes, a Spanish researcher conducted studies in assistance with 13,000 graduates of the University of Navarra. The subjects were recruited between 1999 and 2007 and had no prior history of diabetes. Next, their eating habits were tracked by researchers for a period of almost 5 years.

The survey consisted of a 136 item questionnaire that tracked the frequency of intake of food items during the time period. Participants responded to the questions with their use of fats, dietary supplements and method of cooking. Follow-up questions were sent every 2 years. After the time period, the study found that the participants who followed a diet pattern closely linked with the Mediterranean diet had a lower risk of diabetes. Statistically speaking, the participants with close linkage to the diet had an 83% reduction in the risk. The researchers also found that the diabetic factor was closely linked to one's lifestyle, diet, smoking, etc. and the Mediterranean diet was able to induce significant influence over how the body reacted to attacks by diabetic symptoms.

Chapter 3: Brain

The brain is a vital part of the human body, without which the survival of the rest of the body would be out of the question. The complete elimination of the brain is a farfetched statement; even if the brain suffers from any minor kind of ailment, the whole body suffers and the effects can have lasting implications on the body. Thus it is important that steps be taken that improve one's brain function.

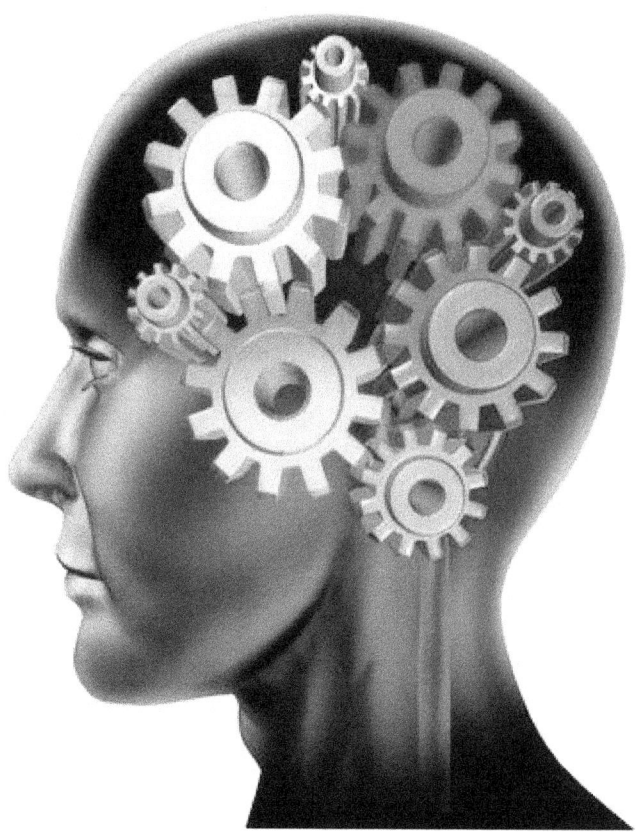

A study was published in the February issue of Archives of Neurology that subjected the Mediterranean diet to tests aimed at finding out its properties in improving brain function. To examine the diet, the data was taken from

Hannah Gardner, Sc.D. at the University of Miami, who conducted a North Manhattan study, targeting 966 participants.

White markers hyper intensities are considered markers of chronic vessel damage. The researchers used the WMHs to obtain an analogical score against Mediterranean diet. The researchers found:

- 11.6% scored 0-2

- 15.8% scored 3

- 23% scored 4

- 23.5% scored 5

- 26.1% scored 6-9

Furthermore, the team discovered that men had higher scores than women along with those who had minimal physical activity throughout the day. Results from the study conclusively indicated that participants who consumed the greatest amount of Mediterranean diet had a lower WMHV count. The connection between brain damage and lifestyle choices like fats, exercise, smoking, etc. was also found, but the one that had the most profound affect was the intake of Mediterranean diet.

Chapter 4: Bones

Everyone knows the importance of healthy bones. Bones are so vital for proper bodily functions that the word itself is used as an idiom to many solid references. But, with the passage of time or sometimes other factors, the quality of a person's bones can fall and he/she can become a victim of conditions like osteoporosis and fractures.

A study published in the Clinical Endocrinology and Metabolism Journal showed that a 2 year long Mediterranean diet along with increased intake of olive oil can decrease the risk of osteoporosis and actually strengthen one's bones. Previously, studies had shown that even though conditions like osteoporosis and bone loss were one the rise in Europe, the number of occurrences in the Mediterranean region were still quite few.

The study consisted of 127 men who were between the ages of 55 and 80 and had been a part of the PREDIMED study (a study center that carries out researches). The volunteers also never had any cardiovascular problem but were diabetics or had risks of diseases like hypertension. The subjects were divided into the following three groups:

i.   A low fat diet group,

ii.   A Mediterranean diet group with Virgin olive oil,

iii.   A Mediterranean diet group with nuts.

The researchers took biological measurements at the start of the study and then after 2 years. The following data was collected:

- Glucose

- Total Cholesterol

- HDL Cholesterol

- Triglycerides

- Osteocalcin

The measurements taken after 2 years showed that intake of Mediterranean diet with olive oil resulted in an increase in the bone-formation units in the body. Supporting results were found with the other Mediterranean group as well and it was concluded that the diet helped in controlling factors that accounted for bone loss.

Recipes

Chapter # 1: Baked Falafel

Makes: 2 servings

Prep time: 20 minutes

Cooking time: 20 minutes

Ready in: 55 minutes

Ingredients:

- ¼ cup chopped onion

- ¼ teaspoon salt

- 1 can garbanzo beans

- ¼ teaspoon baking soda

- ¼ cup freshly chopped parsley

- 1 tablespoon flour

- 3 cloves garlic

- 1 beaten egg

- 2 teaspoon olive oil

- 1 teaspoon cumin, ground

- ¼ teaspoon coriander, ground

Directions:

Wrap the onion in a cheese cloth and squeeze it to a level that all moisture is left out. Set this aside and place the beans, garlic, parsley, coriander, cumin, baking soda and salt in a food processor. Process these until a coarsely pureed mixture is formed and then mix this with the onion. Add in the flour along with the egg and shape the mixture into four patties; let it stand for just 15 minutes. Preheat an oven to 200 degrees Celsius. Heat the olive oil in a large skillet over medium heat and then place the patties in it. Cook them until they are golden brown, which would take about 3 minutes. Finally, transfer the skillet into the preheated oven and bake for 10 minutes.

Chapter # 2: Mediterranean Quinoa Salad

Makes: 4 servings

Prep time: 15 minutes

Cooking time: 20 minutes

Ready in: 35 minutes

Ingredients:

- 2 cubes chicken bouillon
- 2 cups water
- ½ cup kalamata olives
- 1 clove smashed garlic
- ½ cup feta cheese, crumbled
- 1clove garlic
- ¼ cup fresh parsley, chopped
- 1 cup uncooked quinoa
- ¼ cup fresh chives, chopped
- ½ teaspoon salt
- 2 large chicken breasts, cooked
- 2/3 cup lemon juice
- 1 red onion, diced
- 1 tablespoon balsamic vinegar

- ¼ cup olive oil

- 1 large green bell pepper

Directions:

Bring the bouillon cubes, water and garlic to a boil in a large saucepan. Add in the quinoa, reducing the heat to medium, cover and simmer until the quinoa turns tender and absorbs all of the water; this will require 20 minutes. Discard the garlic and pour the quinoa into a large bowl. Stir in the onion, bell pepper, feta cheese, olives, chives, parsley, chicken and salt in the quinoa and drizzle over with balsamic vinegar, olive oil and lemon juice. Stir until the mixture is even and serve while it is still warm.

Chapter # 3: Mediterranean Fish

Makes: 4 servings

Prep time: 15 minutes

Cooking time: 30 minutes

Ready in: 45 minutes

Ingredients:

- ¼ cup capers

- 4, 6 ounce halibut fillets

- ¼ cup olive oil

- 1 tablespoon lemon juice

- 1 tablespoon Greek seasoning

- 1 large tomato

- 1 chopped onion

- 1 kalamata olives jar

- Salt & pepper

Directions:

Preheat an oven to 175 degrees Celsius. Place the halibut fillets on a sheet of aluminum foil and start seasoning it with the Greek seasoning. Combine the onions, olives, tomatoes, olive oil, capers, salt, pepper and lemon juice in a large bowl. Spoon the tomato mixture over the halibut and seal the edges of the foil so as to create a large packet. Place the packet on the baking sheet and bake in the preheated oven for 30 minutes which will be the time taken by the fish to flake using a fork.

Chapter # 4: Roasted Red Pepper Hummus

Makes: 8 servings

Prep time: 15 minutes

Ready in: 1 hour 15 minutes

Ingredients:

- ½ teaspoon ground cumin

- 1 can garbanzo beans, 15 ounce

- ½ teaspoon cayenne pepper

- 1 jar roasted red peppers, 4 ounce

- ¼ teaspoon salt

- 3 tablespoons lemon juice

- 1 tablespoon fresh parsley

- 1 ½ tablespoons tahini

- 1 clove garlic

Directions:

In a food processor or an electric blender, puree the red peppers, chickpeas, tahini, lemon juice, cumin, garlic, cayenne and salt. Process the ingredients using long pulses until a smooth mixture is produced. Scrap off the mixture in between each blend so as to make sure that the mixture is not wasted. Transfer it to a bowl and refrigerate for an hour. (If you want, the hummus may be prepared in advance). Sprinkle the hummus with chopped parsley and finally serve.

Chapter # 5: Greek Lentil Soup

Makes: 4 servings

Prep time: 20 minutes

Cook for: 1 hour

Ready in: 1 hour 20 minutes

Ingredients:

- ¼ cup olive oil
- 2 bay leaves
- 1 pinch crushed dried rosemary
- 8 ounces brown lentils
- 2 bay leaves
- 1 tablespoon tomato paste
- 1 tablespoon minced garlic
- 1 onion, minced
- Salt and black pepper to taste
- 1 large carrot
- 1 teaspoon olive oil
- 1 pinch dried oregano
- 1 quart water
- 1 teaspoon red wine vinegar

Directions:

Place the lentils in a saucepan and pour water in it so that they are covered by at least 1 inch. Bring the water to a boil and allow the lentils to cook until they are satisfactorily tender; this would take about 10 minutes after which you should drain the saucepan. Heat the olive oil over medium heat in another saucepan and add onion, carrots, garlic to it. Cook while stirring it until the onion has turned translucent and softened; this will take 5 minutes. Add in one quart water, lentils, rosemary, oregano and bay leaves. Bring it to a boil and reduce the heat to medium low. Let the mixture simmer for 10 minutes. Add in the tomato paste and season it with salt and pepper; there is no specific amount and you may add as per desire. Cover and simmer until the lentils have developed a soft texture; this may be obtained in 40 minutes, less if perfectly stirred. Add the additional water if the soup is too thick for your taste and finally drizzle with olive oil in combination with red wine before serving.

Chapter 6: Mediterranean Chicken

Makes: 6 servings

Prep time: 20 minutes

Ingredients:

- 2 tablespoons white wine

- 2 teaspoons olive oil

- ½ cup white wine

- 2 teaspoons chopped fresh thyme

- 1 tablespoon chopped fresh basil

- 6 skinless, chicken breast, halved

- 3 cloves garlic

- ½ cup kalamata olives

- ¼ cup fresh parsley

- ½ cup diced onion

- 3 cups tomatoes

- Salt & pepper

Directions:

Heat the olive oil along with 2 tablespoons white wine in a skillet over medium-high heat. Add chicken and sauté for 5 minutes until each side is golden. Remove the chicken from the skillet and put it separately. Sauté the garlic in pan drippings for almost 30 seconds and then add onion, sautéing it again for 3 minutes. Add the tomatoes, bring to a boil, lower the heat afterwards and add ½ cup of white wine, simmering for 10 minutes. Add basil and thyme and let it simmer for another 5 minutes. Return the chicken to the skillet and cover it. Cook the chicken over low heat until it is properly cooked and no longer pink on the inside. Add parsley and olives to the skillet and cook for about a minute; season with salt and pepper.

Chapter 7: Greek Penne & Chicken

Makes: 4 servings

Prep time: 20 minutes

Cook time: 30 minutes

Ready in: 50 minutes

Ingredients:

- 1 package penne pasta, 16 ounces
- ½ cup feta cheese, crumbled
- 3 tablespoons fresh parsley, chopped
- 1 ½ tablespoons butter
- 2 tablespoons lemon juice
- ½ cup chopped red onion
- 1 teaspoon dried oregano
- 2 cloves garlic
- 1 pound boneless chicken breast
- 1 can artichoke
- 1 chopped tomato
- Ground black pepper

Directions:

In a medium sized pot that has boiling water, cook the penne pasta until al dente; drain. Place a large skillet on medium heat and add garlic and onion to it, cooking for 2 minutes. Add chopped chicken and continue to cook, until the color turns golden brown; this will take about 5 minutes. Reduce the heat to medium-low, drain and chop the artichokes. Add these along with feta cheese, chopped tomato, lemon juice, fresh parsley, dried oregano and penne pasta to a large skillet. Cook for 2 to 3 minutes until it is heated thoroughly. Season with black pepper and salt and serve.

Chapter # 8: Pasta Fagioli Soup

Makes: 8 servings

Prep time: 15 minutes

Cook time: 1 hour

Ready in: 1 hour 15 minutes

Ingredients:

- 1 can diced tomatoes, 29 ounces
- 2 cans great Northern beans, 14 ounces
- 8 slices crisp bacon
- 1 tablespoon parsley
- 1 can chopped spinach
- 1 teaspoon garlic powder
- 1 ½ teaspoon salt
- 2 cans chicken broth
- ½ teaspoon ground black pepper
- ½ teaspoon basil, dried
- 1 can tomato sauce
- ½ pound seashell pasta
- 1 tablespoon minced garlic
- 3 cups water

Directions:

In a medium sized, stock pot combine the beans, spinach, tomatoes, broth, sauce, garlic, water, parsley, bacon, salt, pepper, garlic powder and basil. Bring the water to a boil and let it simmer for 40 minutes. Add the pasta and cook for another 10 minutes or until the pasta becomes tender. Ladle the soup into a number of serving bowls and, if desired, sprinkle some cheese on top; finally serve.

Chapter # 9: Italian White Bean Soup

Makes: 4 servings

Prep time: 20 minutes

Cook time: 30 minutes

Ready in: 50 minutes

Ingredients:

- ¼ teaspoon black pepper

- 1 tablespoon vegetable oil

- 1/8 teaspoon dried thyme

- 1 chopped onion

- 2 cups water

- 1 stalk celery

- 1 clove garlic

- 1 bunch of fresh spinach

- 2 cans white kidney beans, 16 ounces

- 1 tablespoon lemon juice

- 1 can chicken broth

Directions:

In a medium sized saucepan heat some oil. Cook the celery and onion in the oil for about 7 minutes or until it turns tender. Now add the garlic and cook it for 30 seconds, continually stirring it. Add in the beans, pepper, chicken broth, 2 cups of water and thyme. Bring the saucepan to a boil and let it simmer afterwards for 15 minutes. With a slotted spoon, remove 2 cups of the vegetable and beans and set it aside. Blend the remaining soup in small batches at low speed until it turns smooth as well. Allow the steam to escape from the blender by removing the center piece. Once the process is complete, pour the soup back into the pot and stir it in the beans reserved earlier. Bring the soup to a boil with occasional stirs. Add the spinach and cook for another minute until the spinach is wilted. Finally stir in the lemon juice, remove from heat and serve with Parmesan cheese on top.

Chapter # 10: Sweet Sausage Marsala

Makes: 6 servings

Prep time: 20 minutes

Cook time: 20 minutes

Ready in: 40 minutes

Ingredients:

- 1 package farfel pasta, 16 ounce

- 1 medium red bell pepper

- 1 pound Italian sausage

- 1 tablespoon Marsala wine

- 1 can Italian-style diced tomatoes, undrained, 14.5 ounces

- 1/3 cup water

- 1 pinch dried oregano

- 1 pinch black pepper

- 1 clove garlic, minced

- ½ large onion, sliced

- 1 green bell pepper

Directions:

Bring a medium sized pot filled with slightly salted water to boil. Cook the pasta in it for 10 minutes; drain. Place the sausages in 1/3 cup of water in a skillet over high heat and cook for 5-8 minutes. Drain afterwards and thinly slice it. Return the sausages to the skillet and stir in the onions, peppers, garlic and Marsala wine. Cook over high heat, stirring frequently and heat until sausage is cooked thoroughly. Stir in the black pepper, oregano and diced tomatoes. Cook for 2 more minutes before removing from heat and serving.

Conclusion

The Mediterranean diet may not be at the top of the diet charts, but it is surely one of the best, most efficient, and at the same time, natural way to bring an overall positive change in your lifestyle. The diet is filled with nutritional goodness that will safeguard you from a variety of illnesses and conditions. Moreover, it isn't only filled with a plethora of health benefits but is also very lively, colorful and delicious to taste. It is a must have for anyone looking to uplift his/her life from a depressing turn of events.

Take care and best of luck!

References

1. http://www.123rf.com/photo_28851211_healthy-vegetable-salad-with-olive-oil-dressing.html?term=mediterranean%20diet

2. http://www.123rf.com/photo_11266323_a-fresh-italian-mozzarella-with-tomato.html?term=mediterranean%20diet

3. http://www.123rf.com/photo_16299043_close-up-of-olive-oil.html?term=mediterranean%20diet

4. http://www.123rf.com/photo_14761332_fish-sea-bass-grilled-with-lemon.html?term=mediterranean%20diet

5. http://www.123rf.com/photo_21637795_illustration-showing-the-circulatory-system.html?term=cardiovascular

6. http://www.123rf.com/photo_16054151_diabetes-concept-glucose-meter-in-hand-and-healthy-organic-food.html?term=diabetes

7. http://www.123rf.com/photo_14119266_intelligence-brain-function-isolated-on-a-white-background-with-gears-and-cog-symbols.html?term=brain

Author Bio

Muhammad Usman is a distinguished medical graduate of Allama Iqbal medical college (AIMC). He is a professional writer who has been in the field for more than 4 years. During this time he has produced 10,000+ articles, blogs and eBooks on various niches related to diseases, health, fitness, nutrition and well-being. He is a regular contributor to several journals related to medicine and surgery. He is the editor of several journals and newspapers.

Our books are available at

1. Amazon.com

2. Barnes and Noble

3. Itunes

4. Kobo

5. Smashwords

6. Google Play Books

Check out some of the other JD-Biz Publishing books

Gardening Series on Amazon

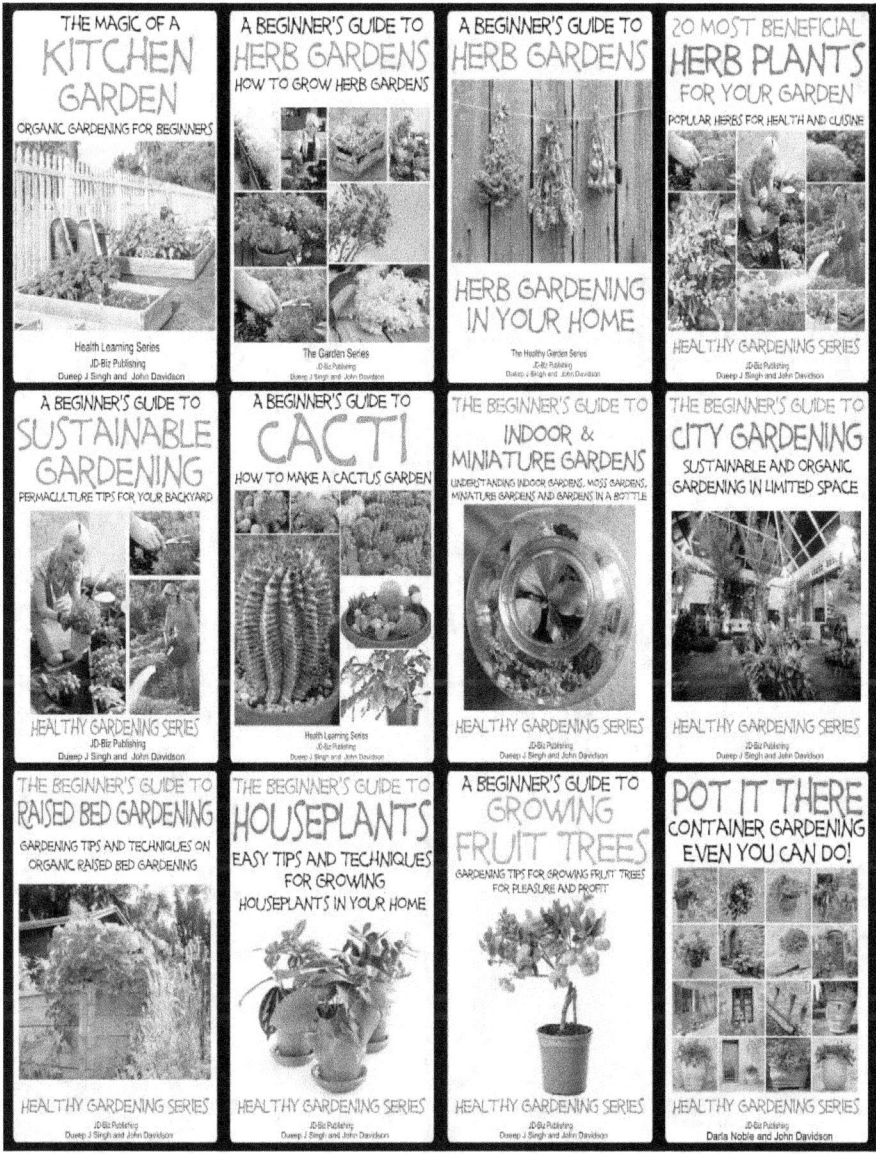

Health Learning Series

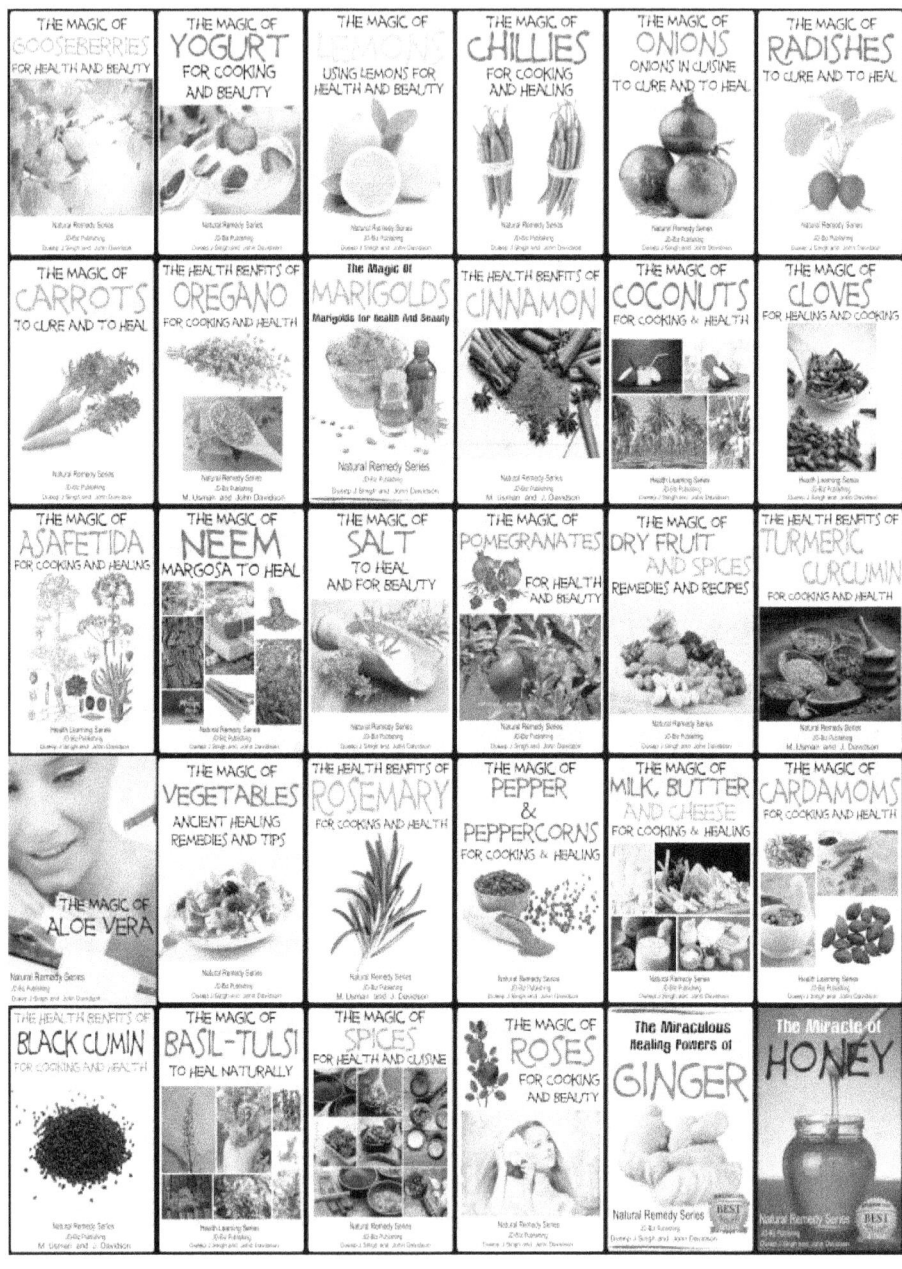

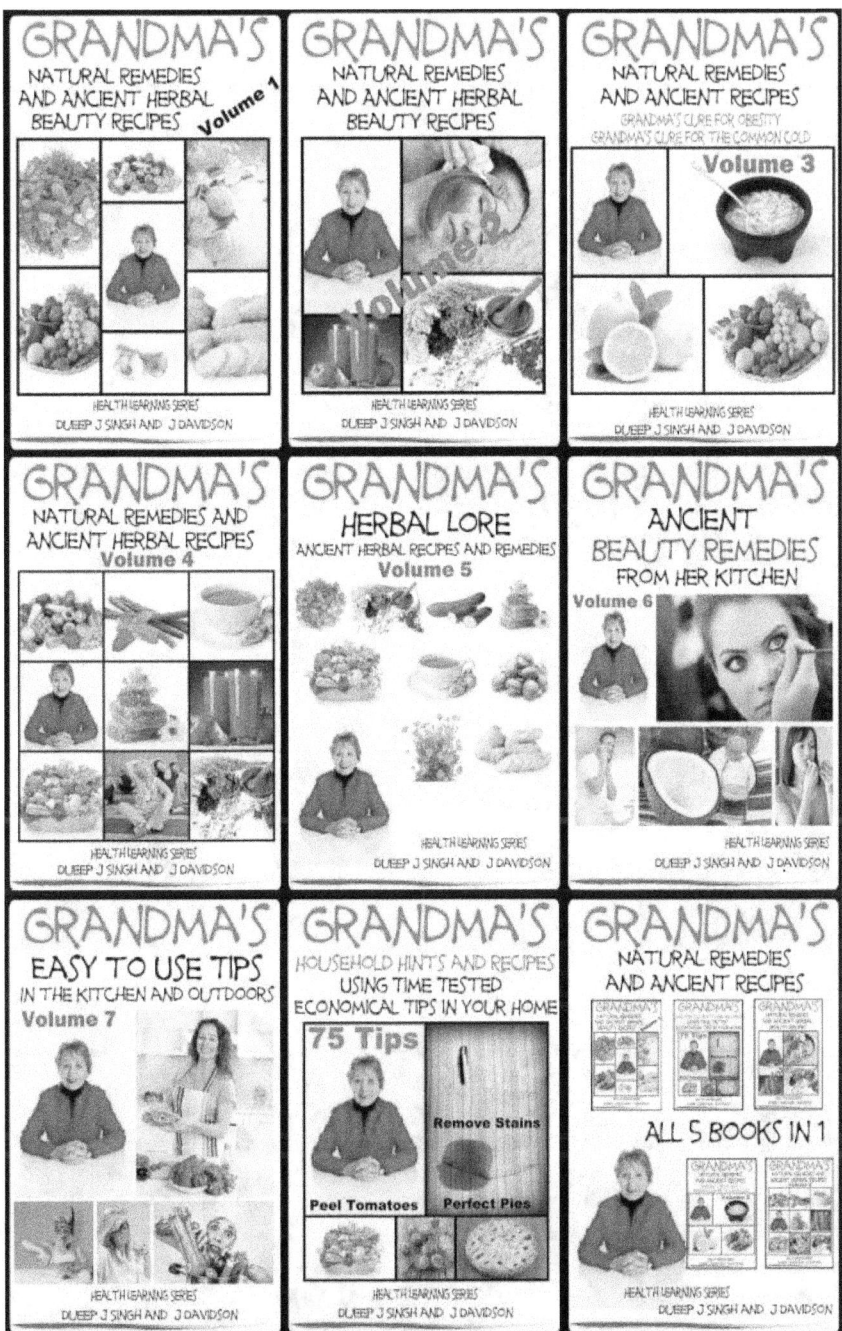

Country Life Books

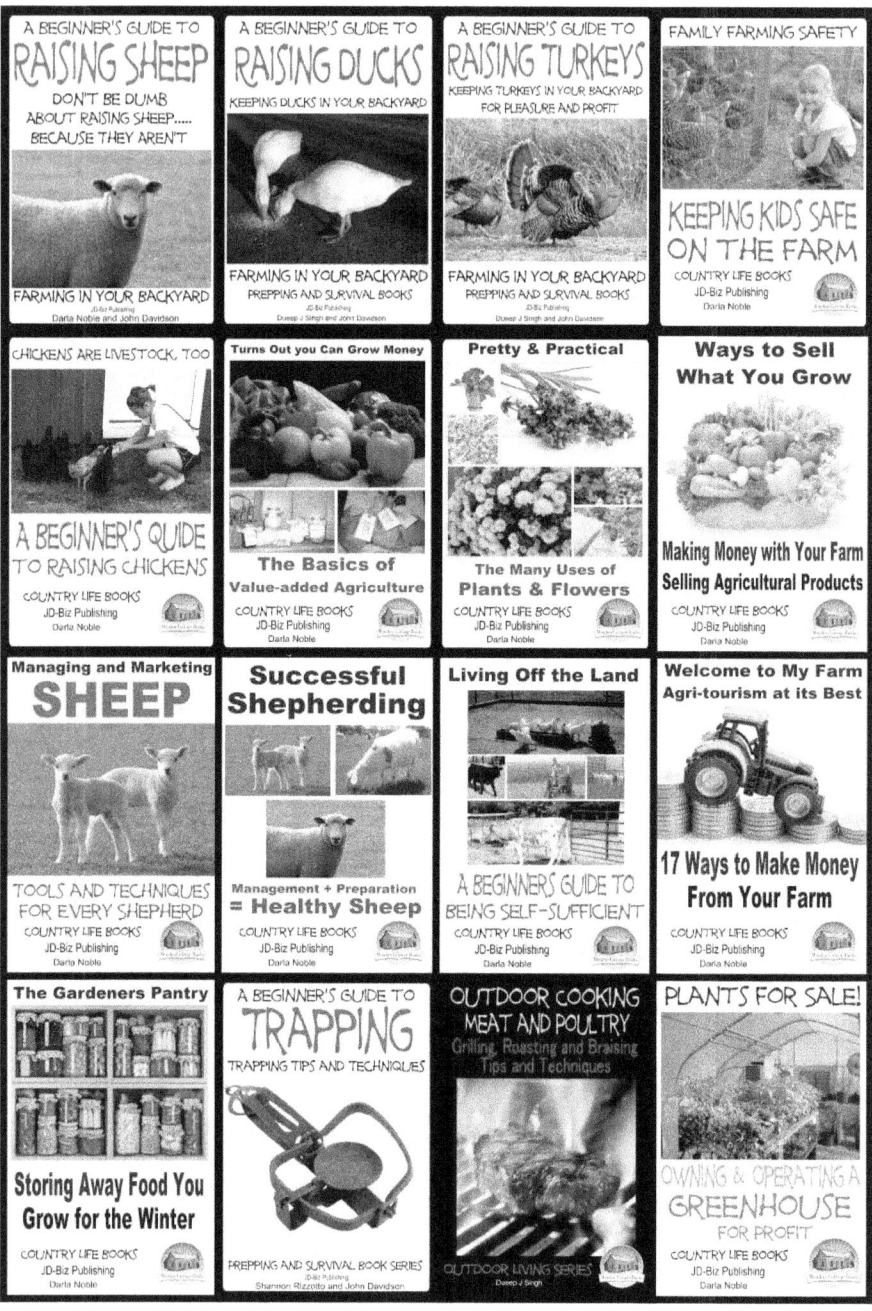

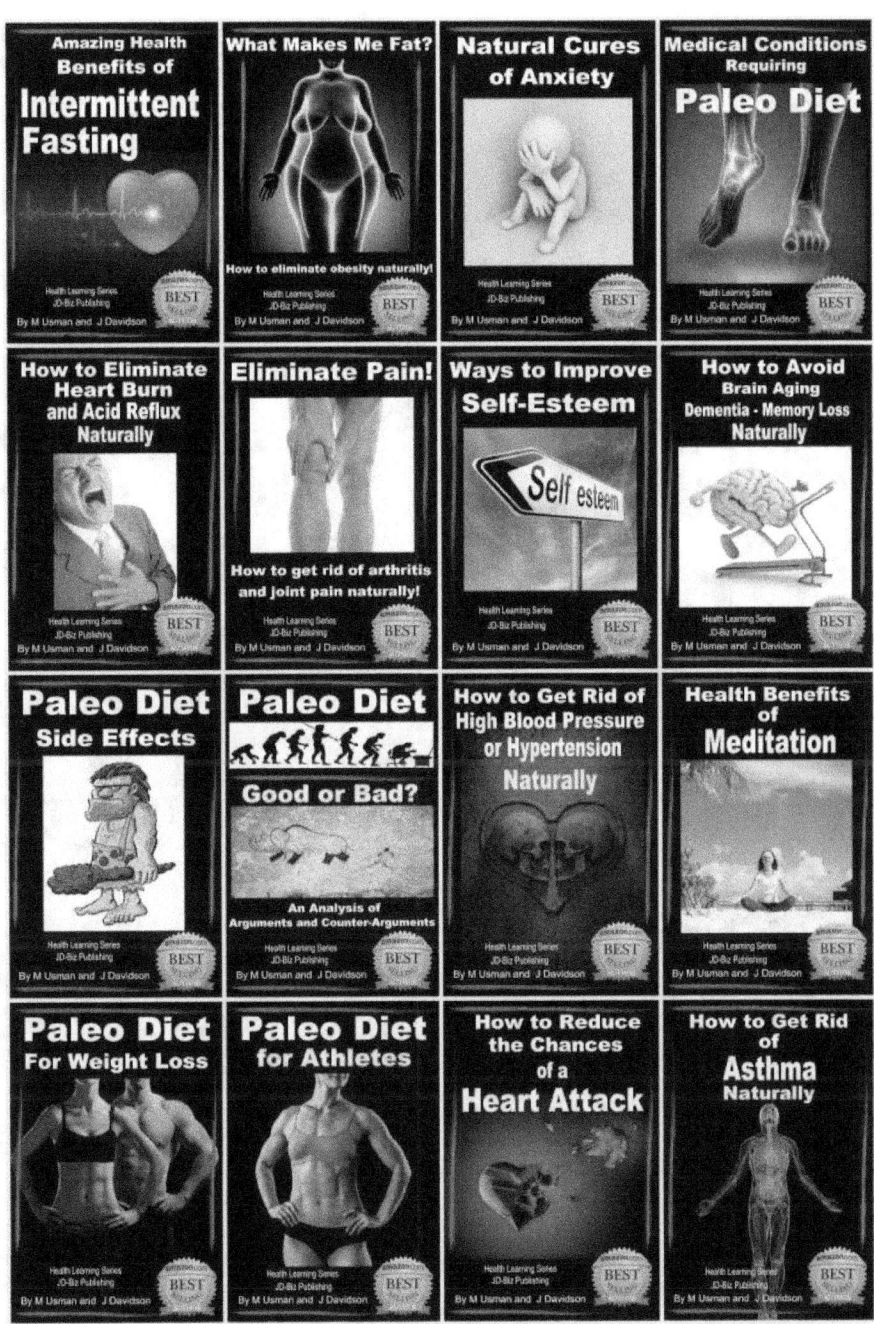

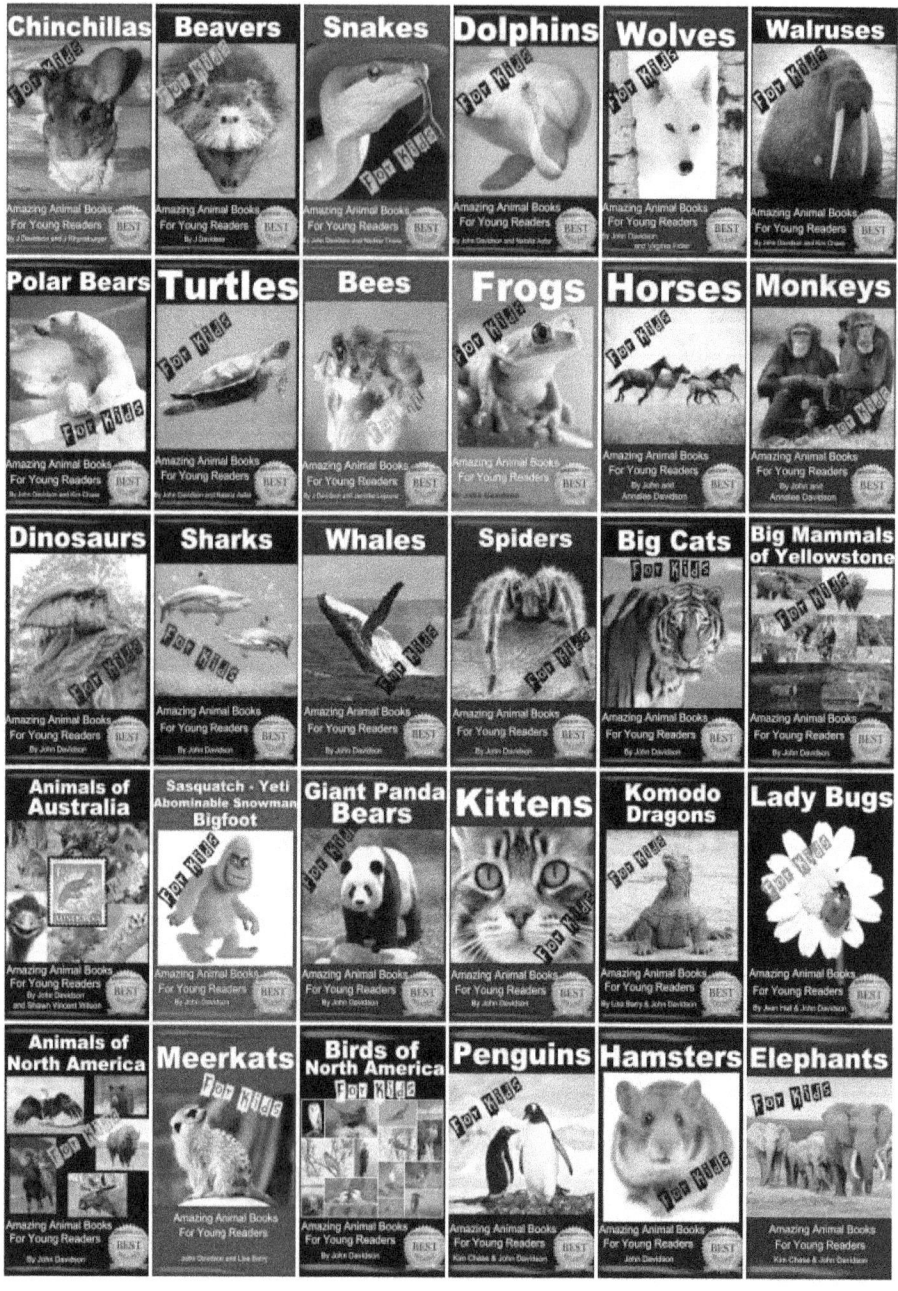

Learn To Draw Series

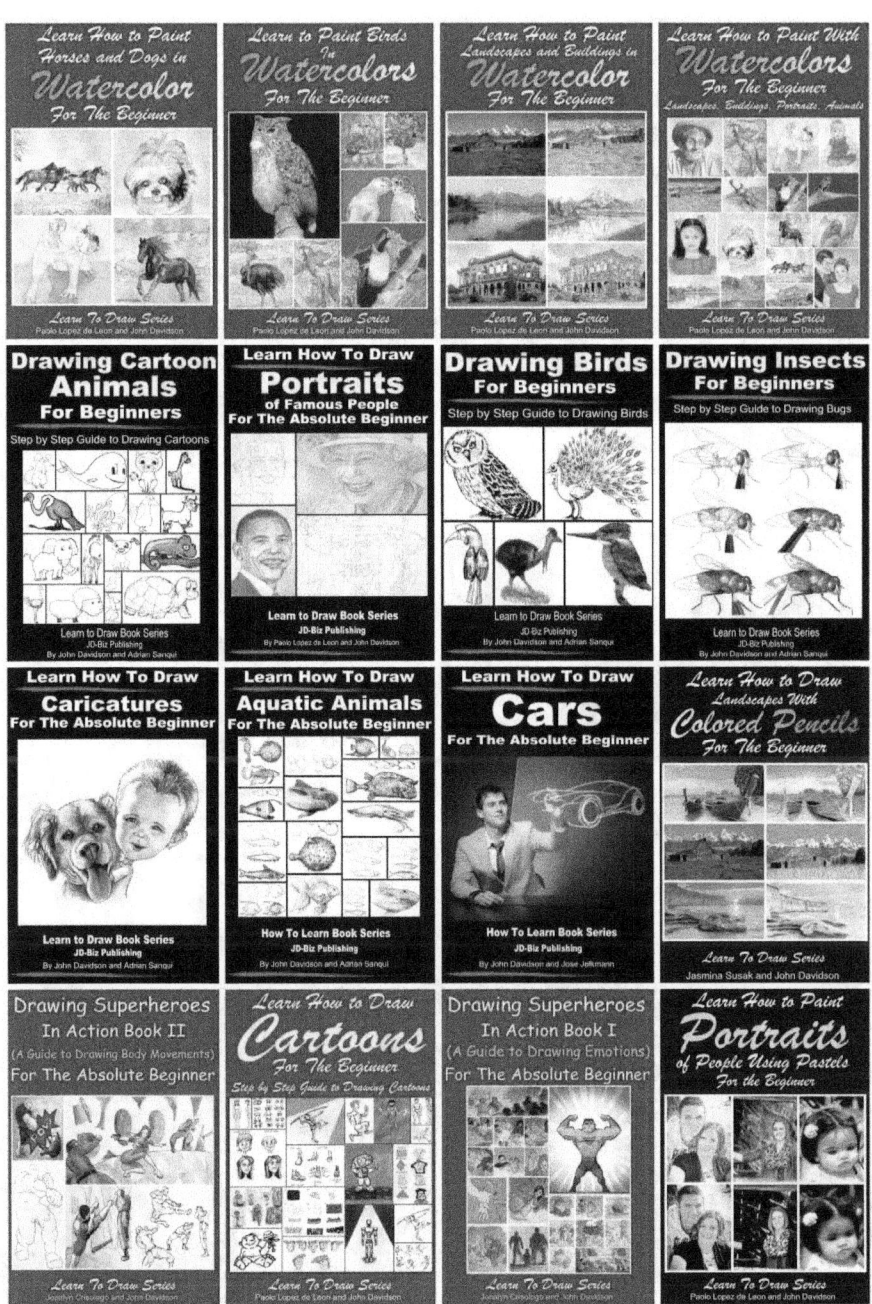

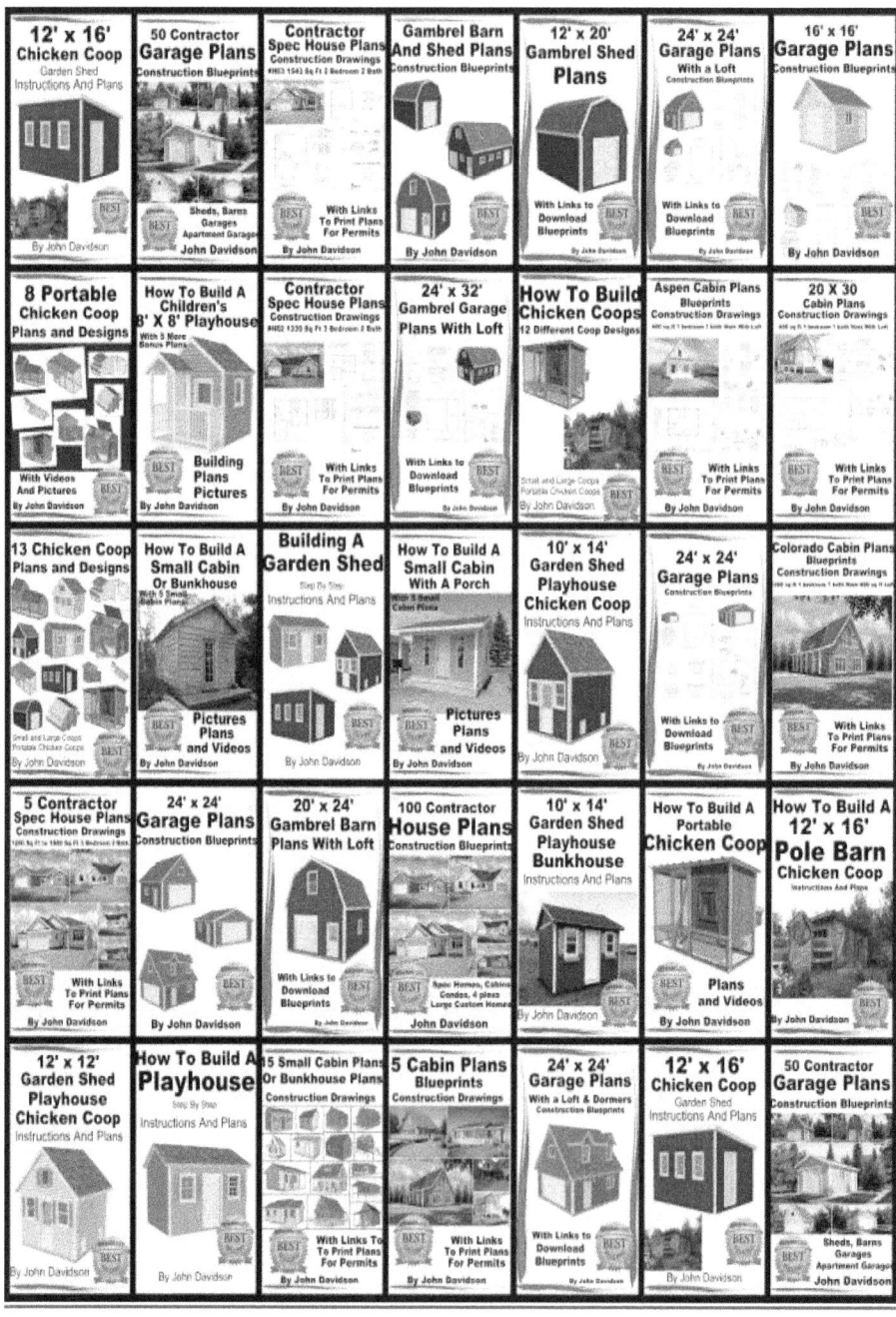

Entrepreneur Book Series

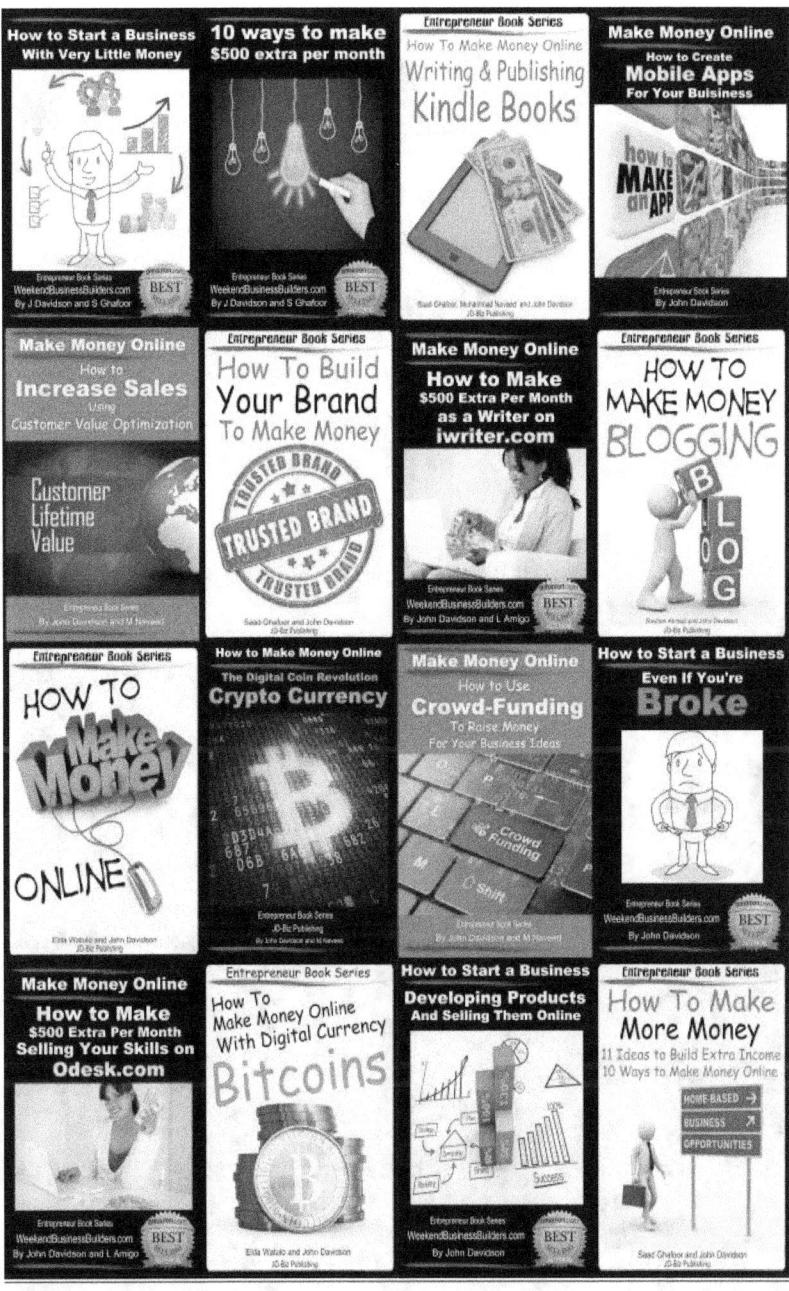

Publisher

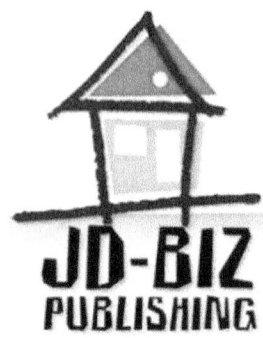

JD-Biz Corp

P O Box 374

Mendon, Utah 84325

http://www.jd-biz.com/

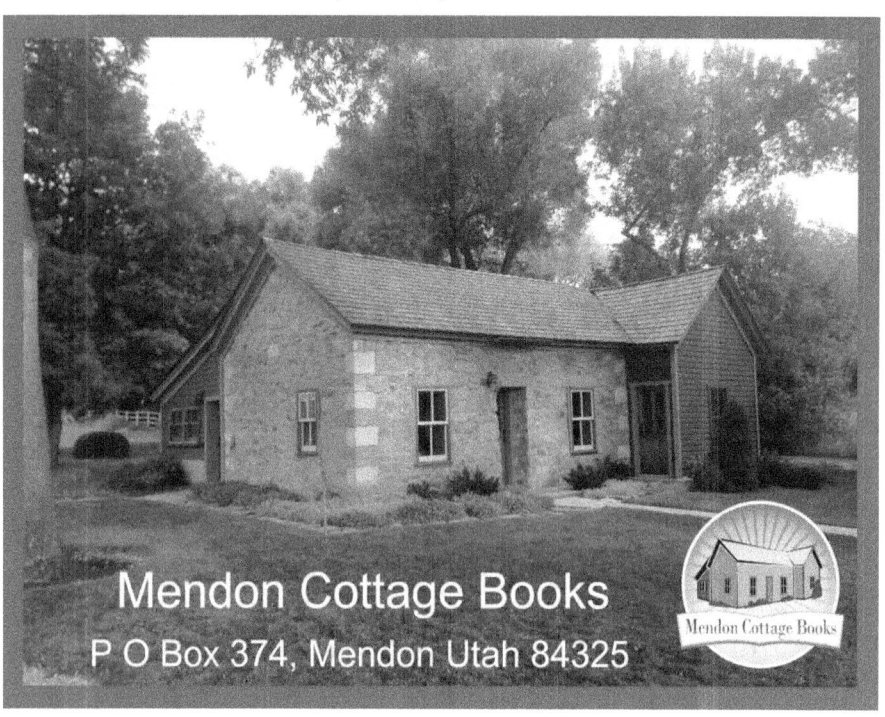

Mendon Cottage Books

P O Box 374, Mendon Utah 84325

www.ingramcontent.com/pod-product-compliance
Lightning Source LLC
Chambersburg PA
CBHW071136280526
45787CB00003B/1300